Zika Virus

When You're

Expecting

Dr. Christopher Maloney, N.D.

DEDICATION

Dedicated to the Zika victims in Brazil and to fearful mothers everywhere. To those who search, that they may find. And use the knowledge to remain Zika free.

CONTENTS

ACKNOWLEDGMENTS

I want to thank the tireless researchers at the World Health Organization, the CDC and all related institutions. Without them, we would have no information about Zika Virus. I would also like to thank my patients, my coworkers, and my family for putting up with me. Finally, I want to thank you for educating yourself about Zika Virus.

Disclaimer

Because of the preliminary nature of research and the changing nature of the Zika viruses, all the ideas presented here may be wrong. Please consult with your local health experts for up-to-date information and rely on them for your health care choices.

PREFACE

Zika virus is big news. We seem to hear daily about small headed babies (microcephaly) and paralyzed victims. It's terrifying, and Zika seemed to come out of nowhere. But Zika has been a threat growing slowly without much publicity. It may be less dangerous than we suspect, but more dangerous if we don't change the way we are approaching its spread.

My goal in this book is to explain what Zika virus is, how it infects, and why we need to change the way we think about how it spreads. By the end of this book, you will know what you need to do to avoid getting Zika, understand how severe Zika occurs, and be better able to protect your family and loved ones.

If you or someone you love is expecting, the reality is that you've been told some partial truths about Zika. Your focus may be on avoiding mosquitoes, when your focus should really be on your previous exposure to similar viruses and the fidelity of your current partner.

Even if they wipe out every mosquito in the Amazon, some travelers will still bring Zika home with them. Not from a mosquito, from a rendezvous with a bitten stranger. Afterward, back in their home countries, the infected will blame the mosquitoes. Zika researchers won't get straightforward answers from victims even when they ask the right questions. Why? Because claiming that you got bitten by a mosquito is much easier than confessing to your partner that it was late, you'd had too much to drink, and you forgot how to say condom in Portuguese (preservativo). Now you're both in quarantine because you've got Zika virus.

Over the last fifty years, despite all our efforts at mosquito control, Zika has spread slowly over the globe, following the same path as Dengue, Yellow Fever, and West Nile Virus. All of these diseases belong to the same family of viruses, and all of them are blamed for their spread by mosquitoes. But all of them may primarily have been passed by human-to-human contact.

We need to rethink about we've defined Zika virus as primarily a mosquito borne disease. Focusing on that one route of transmission leaves us open to transmission and outbreaks "where there shouldn't be any Zika."

Let's work together to keep Zika from all the places it shouldn't be. Pass on your knowledge to your friends and family. Let them know how to be safe. Especially if you're going to have a baby.

1 WHERE DID IT COME FROM?

Somewhere at dusk in post-WWII Uganda out in the swamp a strange ritual is taking place. Local children are slowly climbing a six story tower in the jungle under the watchful eye of white researchers. They stand, waiting silently, their bodies acting as bait for what lurks in the darkness. What horror film is this?

This horror movie set is the Ugandan research station and the researchers are cataloguing mosquito species as well as times and heights of attack. The researchers hired local children as bait, a normal practice in these still-colonial times (Uganda's independence doesn't come until 1962). The tower is in full operation. Six stories of children waiting to be bitten, and mosquito-netted researchers standing near them to snatch the mosquitoes and catalogue them.

The children are the fortunate ones. On one level of the tower sits rhesus monkey 766, bitten over and over again mercilessly by the forty different mosquito species who infest this nasty piece of swampland. The hapless creature is acting as bait for yellow fever research.

Monkey 766 sickens in time, and the researchers draw blood samples to confirm yellow fever. But it isn't yellow fever. No one knows what it is. The swampland where it was found is called overgrown, or Ziika, in the local language. So, dropping the inconvenient extra i, the researchers call the virus Zika virus. It sounds better than "overgrown virus," but it has no more meaning.

As the years pass, Zika is forgotten. Like Rodney Dangerfield, the

Zika virus gets no respect. It is a minor member of the same family as yellow fever, dengue, and West Nile virus (Seventy viruses in all). The symptoms are nearly identical except that Zika is milder. It's like dengue's weaker, slower, and less ferocious kid brother. So no one pays attention to Zika.

Zika isn't tracked, and when occasional epidemics occur in Africa they were noted only by a few researchers. An epidemic of yellow fever-like symptoms in 1954 in Nigeria was documented to be Zika virus and then forgotten. Another Zika outbreak in Indonesia in the 1970's tracks at least thirty hospitalized patients, but the larger medical community ignores it because Dengue and other members of the same family are causing thousands of cases. Zika isn't a public health priority. So when recent news reports on Zika say that less than fourteen human cases were ever reported prior to the current epidemic, they are missing the older reports. By ignoring the past outbreaks of Zika and treating it as a new disease we are panicking ourselves — perhaps unnecessarily.

So how did Zika virus change to become the most recent global scare? To understand that, we need to understand how Zika's family of viruses change over time and infect people.

2 WHAT IS IT?

Zika is part of a family of viruses. You might know some of them: yellow fever, Dengue, West Nile, and the impossible to pronounce Chikungunya virus. The family name is flavivirus, so think of them as different flavors of the same kind of virus. All these flavors live in mosquitoes, humans, and other animals. They are maintained by the transmission of blood and jostle with each other over which gets to infect what parts of the world.

If you catch a flavivirus, chances are you'll feel like you have a cold. You'll get fever, aching joints, and feel tired. Then you'll get better. For most victims, that's the entire disease process. Let me repeat, for almost all victims, getting these viruses is like getting a bad cold.

Only a few patients, just as they're getting better, begin to have serious side effects. With yellow fever, this could include jaundice (turning yellow) and possibly bleeding from your eyes and mouth. Dengue can cause internal bleeding and organ failure. Chikungunya can cause joint pain, damage the nerves, the eyes, or the heart. West Nile virus can cause nerve damage and paralysis. Zika can cause paralysis in adults and microcephaly when the virus attacks the nerves of a growing baby. Again, very few people get these severe symptoms. They are very rare but very concerning because we don't have good treatments once they strike.

Over time the different members of the flavivirus viral family dominate in different regions of the world. So are all the members of the flavivirus family scheming about world domination? Is this a microscopic soap opera where different family members fight for global turf? Or do viruses act without intelligence, dumbly following a mechanical process like the falling of water or growth of crystals? Are we battling a clever microscopic foe or dealing with blind, random genetic selection? We aren't sure, because we aren't even sure viruses are alive.

Let me explain using sex. It's not exact, but more people have experience with sex than immunology.

Remember sex ed class, where a blurry video showed a sperm meeting up with an egg? In a background of junior high school snickers and suppressed giggles, the sperm meets up with the egg and inserts (much laughter here) its genetic material into the egg. As soon as it does that, the sperm has completed its purpose. The egg will take it from here, dividing and becoming a human being or a chicken, depending on which genetic code has been given and what kind of egg it is.

So is the sperm alive? It can't function without the egg. Two sperm can't make a baby. But they do contain genetic material that starts a huge process in motion. Their genetic load is essential for life even if they aren't capable of sustaining it themselves.

A virus is like a sperm. It doesn't function on its own. But it contains genetic material that, when inserted into a cell, starts a cascade of life. All of the cell's machinery is overrun and the purpose of the cell becomes to produce more little viruses. When the cell is full, it bursts, spilling a cascade of viruses out into the body to inject their genetic instructions into other cells.

So is the virus aware of its actions, or is it a mechanical wind-up bit of genetic material that just keeps going and going? Wiser folk than I am are still scratching their heads. We know that viruses develop ways to avoid the immune system, devising clever tricks that look like intelligence. But these may be accidental rather than deliberate because the virus doesn't pass on foolproof genetic material.

It seems like the virus should have an easy life, but there's a problem with being a wandering nomad virus that infects cells for a living. Viruses tend to lack any kind of genetic correcting system. Human DNA has protective mechanisms that make sure that the cell DNA stays the same every time a cell divides. Viruses don't have any way to make sure they stay the same. If a mistake is made, that mistake becomes part of the virus going forward. So viruses mutate at an alarming rate, which can be protective by allowing the virus to avoid capture by the immune system. It can also be destructive, mutating the virus to the point where it no longer replicates well and just goes dormant inside our body's cells (which can also cause us problems – more on that later).

We're all familiar with the mutation rate of the flu. No one expects that this year's flu will be the same as last year's flu. Every year we expect that the flu has mutated so much that we can get it again even though we had it last year. When the flu has a big mutation, we even give it a different name: SARS, Avian influenza, swine flu. Other viruses mutate like the flu, just usually not as fast.

Which brings us to Zika, which isn't one virus. The original Zika virus that infected the rhesus monkey back in 1947 isn't the one we see today. That virus doesn't exist except in laboratory samples. Today there are more than forty variations of Zika virus (currently forty-three and counting). Maybe we should come up with some different names for the different strains rather than sticking with "overgrown virus" for all of them when it wasn't very descriptive in the first place.

The way we can tell it's still Zika virus is that most of the genetic code still matches up. It hasn't jumped over and become West Nile or dengue or another entirely new virus, it's still Zika-ish.

When we track Zika-ish viruses over time, researchers have traced the current Brazilian outbreak strain to Asia, not Africa. Maybe it originated in Africa, but they estimated (based on the level of mutation) that our current Zika-ish viral epidemic was kicking around in Asia for at least fifty years before it made it to Brazil. Think of it as tracking the viral family geneology using genes. The current Zika outbreak is Asian Zika, not African Zika.

It's important to make the distinction, because Asian Zika is the same one that caused the previous explosive outbreaks, first in the Yap Islands in 2007 and later in Fiji and the other Pacific islands. African Zika continues to cause minor periodic outbreaks in Africa, but the Brazilian crisis is caused by the continuing march of a more powerful Asian variation. We saw this storm coming at least ten years ago on the Yap Islands, and it built in force without any larger public health response or media coverage. So the current panic isn't necessarily a sudden mutation in the virus, only an increased media awareness of something that has been happening for some time.

While previously much more mild and likely to be overlooked, the current Asian Zika looks a lot more like the rest of its flavivirus family and now has its own list of serious side effects. Zika has caught up and even bypassed many of its brethren.

While we only have preliminary reports and studies on this Asian

Zika, we can use the history of its viral family members to help us understand how Zika is spread, how and when it causes severe disease, and what is likely to happen with Zika in the future.

3 HOW CAN I GET IT?

If you've read the news reports, the way you avoid Zika is by putting on enough bug spray to kill your neighbor's cat. Oh, and by burning your neighbor's collection of old, used tires which are evidently the most recent weapons of mass mosquito destruction.

But the reality is more complicated. Experts know that Zika has never been spread by mosquitoes alone. Mosquitoes don't travel very far and don't transmit the virus well to their offspring. The female Aedes mosquito travels about four hundred meters in her lifetime, which is twice the distance the tiger mosquito manages. Neither mosquito goes far from the place of her spawning, so trips to other countries and continents aren't on the to-do list. Some experts get around this limitation by citing the "empty tire hypothesis" in which mosquitoes carrying the virus are introduced to a new country using empty tires (more on that in chapter five). But because Zika goes "quiet" for years at a time, mosquitoes alone aren't enough to keep it going (a mosquito lives less than two months).

Because Zika goes "dormant" for decades at a time, experts discuss a "primate vector," which we can picture as some sick monkey troop somewhere in the jungle who carry the Zika virus and occasionally get sick enough to infect the mosquitoes for miles and miles. We know Zika virus can grow in other primates, and it can also affect a range of other animals. Monkeys in Brazil were recently found to be infected by Zika virus. But we don't have proof of a "monkey reservoir" of the disease between outbreaks.

We do know of one primate that passes Zika virus, humans.

Experts have focused previously on mosquito avoidance to control transmission. Then in February 2016 the CDC issued an acknowledgement that sexual transmission did occur and warned Zika infected men to use condoms with their pregnant wives. The CDC had documented the first case of sexual transmission of Zika virus in the U.S. back in 2008, but at that time the connection with birth defects wasn't known so it didn't make the news.

When public health authorities issued the warning to pregnant women it should have been the turning point in how we discuss, approach, and work to control Zika transmission. It was an acknowledgement that Zika virus is a sexually transmitted disease. So women who are not pregnant should always use condoms to avoid getting infected. And men, who have been the only ones documented to transmit the virus sexually, should always use condoms. Having the warning limited to just pregnant women will help protect their infants but won't prevent the spread of Zika.

If we're truly interested in controlling Zika, it would seem that we should add condoms to the conventional list of controls: 1) avoid getting bitten, 2) get rid of tires, and 3) avoid having unprotected sex with any recently infected with Zika.

But even those cautions might not be enough. Zika virus has been found in both the saliva and the urine of infected individuals, where it can continue for months after the infection. We don't have any saliva-only or urine-only proven cases, but there is a possibility that Zika is passed via respiratory droplets. That raises the possibility of food borne transmission or transmission via coughing or sneezing. If Zika is passed by saliva, then mosquitoes are just a distraction from what is a primarily a human-to-human disease. But, until we have conclusive evidence that saliva alone is infectious (rather than just contains fragments of the virus), we need to focus on the known concerns.

At this point, we know that any type of sexual encounter (oral, anal, or vaginal) may spread the virus in addition to any mosquito bites you may receive. So avoiding mosquitoes and being safe are what you need to avoid getting the Zika virus.

1)   Avoid getting bitten by mosquitoes.

2)   Avoid unprotected sex.

4 HAVE I ALREADY HAD IT?

Here's the good news: you may already have had the Zika Virus and not known it. If you did, you likely have lifelong immunity.

Consider the following scenario. You may or may not remember getting a mosquito bite. About a week later, you felt ill, perhaps with a headache. Then you came down with a fever, your joints hurt, and you were sick for about a week. There you go. That could have been Zika. Or the flu. Or a cold. Or any of a wide range of other illnesses. The point is the vast majority of people who get Zika may not even know they had anything more than a cold.

But let's say for argument's sake you've never even had a bad cold. You may still have had Zika and not known it. It's possible you were infected with Zika and never had any symptoms. An infectious disease panel says eighty percent of those infected with Zika never get any symptoms. The World Health Organization puts the number much lower, but they still estimate at least a quarter of people who come down with Zika show no symptoms.

If you don't show any symptoms, that doesn't mean you didn't get the virus. Our immune system is perfectly capable of recognizing a viral intruder, building a defending army, and defeating that intruder without any symptoms showing up. Only when the intruder is new and nasty does it have a chance of getting a foothold strong enough that the body has to generate physical symptoms to make us give our full attention to the illness. Once that initial illness is resolved, our body keeps memory cells circulating that will make the next attack from that virus short and probably symptom-free.

Now, if you don't show symptoms of Zika, are you still infectious? Possibly. Both the saliva and the urine of infected individuals continues to dump out the virus well after the person has gotten over any Zika symptoms. So simply because a person hasn't had Zika symptoms in the last month doesn't mean they aren't infectious. They may have had the virus, be infectious now, and not know it. So Zika may sit quietly in a population for years without anyone really noticing.

But don't the recent Zika outbreaks show that everyone is getting Zika all at once? Maybe. Researchers of the previous outbreaks recorded both patients with symptoms and anyone that had an immune response to Zika virus. They reported both as being part of the current outbreak, assuming that any immune response meant the person had the illness recently.

But patients with an immune response to Zika virus might have been infected years previously. In countries where there has been no major Zika outbreak researchers tracking Zika found about five percent of the population had antibodies to the Zika virus. So researchers who count both symptomatic patients and anyone who has an immune response may make the outbreaks appear worse and more sudden than they are.

Let's use you as an example of how you might mistakenly show up as part of a Zika outbreak. If you've been exposed to Zika at any point, you'll show up positive for an immune response because your memory cells will remember that virus and produce a few anti-Zika antibodies to be ready in the future. Since we don't test most people for Zika unless there's an outbreak, there's no way your doctor would know you'd had it. So five years from now if there's an outbreak of Zika in your community, you'd likely be tested for the first time and be included as a victim of that outbreak.

So, should we all get tested to see if we have been exposed to Zika? No. Right now testing for Zika is difficult because it's hard to tell Zika apart from the other flaviviruses, especially dengue. Testing is currently only being done in major public health centers and the best results seem to be in the first three days after an active infection. We need to make sure those who really need the tests get them. Currently even pregnant women who test positive for Zika but who don't have symptoms or birth complications are not reported to public health officials.

5 HOW IS IT SPREAD?

For pregnant mothers and anyone who knows them, the Zika scare has likely led to a lot of extra insect repellent being given at baby showers. It's also caused a lot of extra calls to the doctor over mosquito bites. Because we all know that Zika virus is spread by mosquitoes.

Except, what we all know is wrong. The Zika virus is not spread by mosquitoes. It's spread by humans.

I hope that got your attention, because if anyone has followed the spread of Zika, you've been inundated by the mantra of "mosquito spread disease."

Yes, both mosquitoes and humans are carriers of Zika. Yes, mosquitoes are the way that local areas get saturated with cases of Zika as the local house mosquitoes pass infected blood from neighbor to neighbor. But if you want to spread the virus to a new area, say from Brazil to France, it's not going to be spread by mosquitoes. It's going to be spread by humans. This may seem like a nit-picky little detail but it makes a huge difference. Humans travel farther and are not restricted by temperature extremes. So thinking about humans as the spreading agent determines how far Zika can travel and who should be concerned about getting infected.

It's likely that humans have always been responsible for the spread of Zika. Let's go back in time. I want to show you a map, but first I want to talk a bit more about the mosquitoes that are held responsible for spreading Zika virus.

If you've been obsessing about Zika virus, you know that there are two species of mosquito that primarily spread the infection. The Aedes female mosquito travels less than four hundred meters from her place of birth. The other species we know that can harbor Zika, called a tiger mosquito, travels less than 200 meters in her life. The female mosquito will eat near where she was born, and she'll likely return to the swamp that birthed her to lay her eggs. She doesn't go on holiday, and she isn't a world traveler. Keep that in mind as you look at the following map of the spread of the Zika virus over time in Africa.

See the jumps? Those arrows point to major leaps as the virus crosses half the African continent. Follow one arrow, and it appears that a mosquito decided to travel from Uganda to Malaysia.

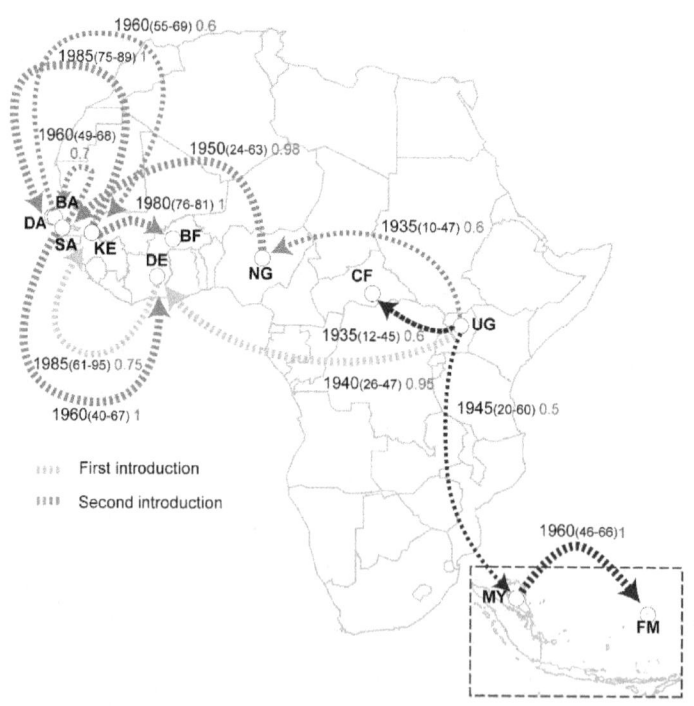

Faye O, Freire CCM, Iamarino A, Faye O, de Oliveira JVC, Diallo M, et al. (2014) Molecular Evolution of Zika Virus during Its Emergence in the 20th Century. PLoS Negl Trop Dis8(1): e2636. https://doi.org/10.1371/journal.pntd.0002636 Creative Commons Attribution License.

The Empty Tire Model

Ah, but couldn't that mosquito been smuggled aboard a ship? Or couldn't it have hidden its eggs in something and sent them to Malaysia? The most popular version of this idea is the "empty tire" model. Tires with water in them are shipped around the world, traveling to foreign climes and bringing mosquitoes with them. The mosquito eggs can remain viable even when dried out for up to eight months. The transfer of mosquitoes via ships and tires can and does happen (tires make great traps for mosquitoes), but the explosive nature of the Zika epidemics would necessitate some sort of mass mosquito invasion.

Since tire transfer is the dominant medical model for the spread of Zika, let's explore the empty tire concept. Imagine, if you will, a group of female mosquitoes all reading the shipping news and all deciding to lay their eggs in the tires of one ship bound for Malaysia. Or perhaps it's a ship full of old tires that were trucked from Uganda to the coast. Some kind of old tire exchange program.

So, following the transfer of many mosquito eggs, the ship docks in Malaysia during a sudden rainstorm that rehydrates all the dried mosquito eggs. The mosquitoes all simultaneously begin to grow, a process that takes seven to ten days.

We'll assume that all the eggs were infected with Zika virus, though we have no research to confirm that Zika virus can be passed down from a mother mosquito to her child. Studies on transmission of dengue, which is so close to Zika in can lead to false positive lab tests, shows about fifteen percent of baby mosquitoes can transmit dengue. But we'll assume a hundred percent transfer of Zika virus for our model.

If the baby mosquitoes didn't have Zika already in them, they would have to grow up and bite a Zika infected sailor before they could get it. That scenario might be more likely, but it slows our epidemic. The Zika virus takes from four to fourteen days from the time an adult mosquito bites an infected sailor to when the Zika virus is present in the adult mosquito's saliva. So it would be roughly half a mosquito's life before it became infectious to humans. Depending on the mosquito, the infectiousness of its saliva could be low. In the current epidemic, researchers have found that mosquitoes aren't very good at passing on the virus.

But we're going to ignore the need to bite any humans because all of our mosquitoes are Zika-ready from birth. They buzz out of our cargo of old tires ready to start the epidemic. Since the mosquitoes only fly about four hundred meters from their home ship, if mosquitoes alone were responsible for the spread of Zika we would expect to see a progressive outbreak of human Zika cases from the docks outward. At that point, because the original mosquitoes haven't left their ship, the virus is spread from mosquito to human to new local house mosquitoes further inland, which slows things considerably. The progress would be a week for human illness, followed by at another two weeks before the biting mosquitoes have infectious saliva. The disease would move gradually inland over months, with inland cases showing up well after the dock workers' infections had resolved. A researcher should be able to draw rings around the original infection and show the origin of the disease outbreak (even pinpoint the infected ship). Based on mosquito flight patterns, we could also measure how far we'd expect Zika virus to have spread over a certain period of time as it moves through the mosquito population.

Instead, during the 2007 outbreak seventy percent of the Yap islanders experiencing the infection in a single year. It wasn't progressive, it was rapid. The tire model doesn't explain the rapidity of the outbreak very well.

Another issue with the empty tire model is that once a mosquito species had taken the time to invade all the way to the Yap Islands, we would expect to see prolonged and continual illness. Instead, we see an outbreaks followed by whole periods of "silence" when Zika doesn't seem to cause any widespread illness. Then, suddenly, it will again strike a wide group of the population seemingly all at once. The mosquitoes didn't leave after invading, they didn't dwindle to nothing and suddenly recur. They stayed and continued to feast, but no one got sick.

One could argue that droughts caused the mosquito populations to dwindle, but there is no evidence that Zika infection follows drought patterns. Researchers have found that too much rain can wash away eggs and larvae, so that mosquitoes are heaviest in the post-monsoon season when water becomes more stagnant. During the current Brazilian epidemic, experts think drought-like conditions may have worsened the mosquito problem because humans were storing more stagnant water indoors where the mosquitoes could breed.

Previous Zika outbreaks might have supported the empty tire

model, but the current epidemic is happening far too quickly to allow for the leisurely spread of mosquito laden tires. In 2015, Zika cases were found in Samoa, the Solomon Islands, Fiji, and Vanatu, almost simultaneously. Experts got around the rapidity of the spread by calling the cases "autochthonous," meaning that they spontaneously arose from local native mosquitoes rather than being transferred by empty tires. In other words, these Zika outbreaks occurred as a result of locally sick monkeys coincidentally infecting mosquitoes at the same time that outbreaks were occurring on other islands. While I love the term autochthonous, it still seems unlikely that these outbreaks had no connection to the Brazilian outbreak.

In Brazil, Zika spread across the whole country in three months, barely time for two generations of mosquitoes to reach the age of being infectious. By September 2015, Columbia reported almost four thousand cases. By December 2015, Zika had spread through all of Central America. But again, public health authorities said that many of these cases were local, native "autochthonous" cases, not spread from Brazil. The only viral testing done showed a 99% genetic match between the Brazilian cases and the previous 2013 epidemic in French Polynesia. But acknowledging that the spread of Zika could happen so quickly means abandoning completely the empty tire model of Zika transmission.

The Unwary, Horny Traveler Model

There's another hypothesis that is simpler than the empty tire model of the spread of Zika virus. Call it the "unwary horny traveler" model of transmission. Let's use the Uganda to Malaysia jump again. A traveler gets bitten by a mosquito and infected with Zika virus in

Uganda. He then travels to Malaysia for business. There he has unprotected sex with several people. They all get Zika from him and get sick, but only after they've been with other people. Later, some of the sick people are bitten by local house mosquitoes, who help maintain the virus locally by giving it to family members and anyone who lives within four hundred meters. Friends come to visit, getting bitten and bringing the virus with them to spread to their own local mosquito colonies. Notice in this model, it is the human, not the mosquito, who is responsible for spreading the virus. The mosquito maintains it and infects family and friends who visit, but the movement of the virus from town to town and country to country is entirely due to human carriers.

Comparing the mosquito model to the human model, it seems more likely new outbreaks get their start from other humans rather than waiting for the spread of mosquitoes. It was the humans getting bitten that infected the local mosquitoes, who then helped maintain the virus in their local area. To say that the mosquitoes caused the outbreak ignores the reality that they weren't able to move rapidly enough to have that kind of impact. Humans infect the mosquitoes first, not the other way around.

If it's an easier explanation that humans spread Zika, why are we focused on the mosquitoes? It limits our vulnerability to Zika virus, and gives those of us outside the "Zika mosquito zones" a false sense of security. It also slows the concern we'd all feel about the idea that anyone, anywhere in the world, could be a carrier of Zika virus. He or she may not know they're a carrier, having never experienced any symptoms because their immune system was so efficient at dealing with the virus. But the carrier may still be able to transfer the virus to others.

So, is there any other model for this sort of human-borne epidemic? Yes. We have the model that we see every year. A flu comes into the community. It goes through the community rapidly, and is over once most of those susceptible have had it. Then it goes away again, going "silent" until the next mutation when it comes back around. But using that model means acknowledging that it is humans, not mosquitoes, that are the primary cause of the spread of the Zika virus.

If you read all the reports about Zika, most experts do try to combine some human transmission with mosquitoes. But they always fall back on mosquitoes, not the humans, as the reason for the illness.

"How did you get Zika?" The experts might try to answer an angry man who has been wearing insecticide like an extra coat for weeks. "Imagine a person with Zika comes to town and gets bitten," they say. "The mosquitoes incubate the virus and spread it through town." And mosquitoes certainly do maintain the virus locally, so it's not a lie. It's just a misdirection. It's a lot easier to blame mosquitoes than to say something along the lines of, "a stranger came to town and had unprotected sex with your unfaithful girlfriend. She infected you, and that's how you got Zika." All over the world, mosquitoes are being blamed for all sorts of diseases. It's a lot easier than coming clean about human behavior.

So how do you get Zika? Go to an endemic area and live in the house next to someone with Zika. Then use no mosquito netting or other precautions and allow yourself to be bitten by a mosquito that can carry the virus. Currently both of the known species are limited to the southern United States and southern climes throughout the world. In other words, if you believe the mosquito based model, you have no chance of getting Zika unless there are mosquitoes.

Or you could have unprotected sex (straight or otherwise) with someone who has been infected with Zika. That can happen anywhere in the world, and the person you get Zika from may not know they are infectious. It's a lot less reassuring, but we need to be aware of that model of Zika transfer.

The bottom line is that for anyone not currently living in a mosquito-ridden area the only way to get the virus is by swapping body fluids with another human being. If you live in a mosquito-ridden area, avoid getting bitten (and maybe set up a mosquito trap or two). But also don't swap body fluids with strangers regardless of where you live. Which should be common sense, but doesn't seem as common as it should be.

6 MOSQUITOES, SEX, AND BLOOD

The Zika virus officially became a sexually transmitted disease in the U.S. in 2008 when the CDC documented a health care worker infecting his wife with Zika virus far from any infectious mosquitoes.

So why, almost a decade later, are we surprised that Zika virus is transmitted sexually? Public health efforts continue to focus on mosquitoes, when the spread of Zika may have always been via human transmission. Don't get me wrong, mosquitoes maintain Zika, they just don't spread it (much) – people do.

Mosquitoes can pass Zika virus. So can having unprotected sex. But what these share is blood. Not a lot, just a little blood is enough to transmit the virus. Until we know for certain that saliva alone can transmit Zika virus, avoid sharing blood with others.

It may not be obvious just how much of a problem this could be until we start thinking about the world blood supply available for transfusions during surgeries. In a pregnancy that might end in complications, a blood transfusion might be necessary. Currently no simple lab screen is available for testing blood for Zika, and areas with Zika outbreaks have stopped collecting blood until testing can be developed. Several cases of Zika infections from infected blood have already been reported in Brazil. Right now if you get a transfusion, it hasn't been tested to be clean of Zika virus.

Beyond surgical concerns, a blood-borne disease becomes a sexually transmitted disease. Currently only pregnant women are getting the message that their bedroom behavior can put the unborn infant at risk. It isn't just them, it's everyone. If you have unprotected sex and become a Zika carrier, you can bring Zika back to the pregnant women in your community and give it to them through local mosquito maintenance.

The current mosquitoes known to harbor Zika virus are in the southern climes, but we have no information on whether other mosquitoes or animals like ticks or black flies might also carry and transmit the virus. If we're looking at a recent bite where the animal still has infected blood in its abdomen, then it is a very real concern that Zika could be passed. Other members of Zika's viral family can transmit using birds, bats, ticks, and other animals as a reservoir. No research on Zika exists to let us know how far its range may be expanded by other animal species traveling from place to place.

Another aspect of being blood-borne is that human behaviors, including IV drug use, can spread the virus without any mosquito involvement. Again, we have no information on the extent of Zika virus in IV drug users, but we know that accidental needle sticks can transmit the virus to researchers.

Perhaps as high as eighty percent of human-to-human transmission may go undetected. A person might be infected without symptoms and might transmit the disease to another person who gets it, but also who doesn't develop the disease. Individuals may be non-symptomatic carriers of the disease for at least two months, which is as long as the entire lifecycle of a carrying mosquito. Since we haven't been looking for it, we have likely missed the relative frequency of human-to-human transmissions. "Silent" transmission may be much more common than we suspect.

Is Zika unique among the flaviviruses in its ability to be

transmitted via the blood from human to human? No. Zika isn't the first flavivirus to have possible human-to-human transmission recorded. West Nile virus has been transferred via breast milk, blood transfusions, and from mother to unborn child. Chikungunya virus has been found in infectious levels in the blood supply. Dengue can be passed directly from organ donor to recipient. In 2009 doctors documented that yellow fever can transmit directly from mother to child.

But, despite documented transmission between humans, all of the focus on the flaviviruses has been on their transmission by mosquitoes. It's been reasonable, because mosquitoes are far more efficient at maintaining an illness within an area. But it's time to openly look at blood borne human-to-human transmission if we want any hope of slowing the spread of these illnesses to new regions and countries.

7 BIRTH DEFECTS

Since avoidance doesn't always work, we need to consider the worst case scenario. So you're pregnant, you've been bitten (or naughty), and you come down with Zika virus. You have all the symptoms and they confirm it is Zika virus at a CDC lab within three days of your infection. That's it. You've doomed your child, right?

Not necessarily. While the reports from Brazil are alarming, we don't know for certain that Zika virus is the cause. Other less alarming causes like alcohol use or local environmental factors might be the true culprits.

But it doesn't look good for Zika. Autopsies and brain fluid have found Zika virus in the brains of the babies. The Zika virus seems to prefer to spread through nerve tissue, which makes the brain a ripe target once it gets there.

So how likely is your baby to be borne with a small head (microcephaly) as a result? The best information we have on the last outbreak in French Polynesia puts the risk to the child at around one percent. The most dramatic statistical estimates from Brazil might raise the risk as high as 13%, but those are more questionable numbers.

In other words, in the worst case scenario a child infected with Zika still has an extremely good chance of being born normally. Chances are also very good that the child could catch Zika from the infected mother, but that doesn't necessarily mean the child is at risk for Guillain-Barré syndrome (see next chapter).

We currently don't have longer term, reliable information on the outbreak in Brazil. Reporting of microcephaly was not required by the Brazilian authorities before the most recent outbreak. So the previous official reported rate of microcephaly in Brazil was at least four times lower than the reported U.S. rate. Just keep in mind we are looking at funny statistics when we see the explosion in Brazilian microcephaly.

But the spike of cases in Brazil is still much higher than one would expect, and the infants show Zika virus in their brains on autopsy. In several cases the Brazilian mothers did not show a Zika virus infection but their microcephalic children did. Clearly there is a connection. But that doesn't mean that Zika alone is causing the problem.

During the same time as the Brazilian Zika epidemic, the closely related dengue and chikungunya viruses were also moving through the same population. While chikungunya is also a relative newcomer, dengue has been around for some time. And dengue co-infection could be part of the cause for the microcephalic children.

Dengue, like Zika, is a flavivirus. They are so closely related that lab testing for antibodies have difficulty telling them apart. The antibodies "cross-react" attacking one or the other almost as if they are the same virus. Most people get dengue and recover in a week. But a few do not. At particular risk are newborns, who get dengue from their mothers. The infants most at risk are those whose mothers have also been previously infected with a different strain of dengue virus.

Currently there are four different strains of dengue, helpfully called 1, 2, 3, and 4. Being infected with one strain gives you lifelong immunity to that strain, but not the others. Getting infected with a second strain of dengue isn't good. It makes it more likely for an adult to have severe dengue side effects (Guillain-Barré) and for a pregnant mother's unborn infant to have severe birth defects.

Why does the second dengue infection increase the risk of severe disease? In studies of immune response to the flavivirus family, researchers found that a previous infection could cause the body to generate more of an immune response to that past infection than the current one. This response is called an "anamnesia" response, the opposite of amnesia, which is forgetting. In this case the body remembers the past infection too well and overreacts by sending out a flood of antibodies to fight the past infection.

The Trojan Horse Model

It might be easier to understand the response to two different dengue strains if we use two different members of the flavivirus family. I'll use dengue and Zika. If a person had dengue, for example, the immune response against dengue could be activated if the person later got infected with Zika Virus. Not only could the dengue immune response be triggered, it would be triggered at a much higher level than the body's immune response to the Zika virus itself. Because these viruses look so similar to the body, the immune memory cells for dengue would pull out all the stops and mount a tremendous counterattack against what they think is another attack of dengue. Unfortunately for the person involved, all those dengue antibodies wouldn't kill the Zika virus. They would surround the virus, enveloping it, but wouldn't be able to destroy it. Then other immune cells, the cleanup crew, would come and engulf the supposedly dead virus and antibodies. Once inside the immune cell, the Zika virus would break free and use the immune cell as a factory to make more viruses. So the dengue immune response could act to increase the severity of the Zika infection by drawing the still-active Zika virus into the immune system's cleanup cells. The Zika virus hides inside the dengue antibodies, emerging to invade the cells from within in a Trojan Horse model.

We know this is what happens when two different strains of dengue attack a pregnant mother. Because an unborn infant is dependent on its mother's immune system, a secondary dengue infection can be particularly serious. The mother's previously infected immune system attaches onto the new strain of dengue using antibodies that would have killed the other strain of dengue. In this case the immune system of the mother ends up creating a Trojan horse, surrounding the virus but keeping it alive until it reaches the infant. Since the virus isn't dead, it releases its genetic instructions into the infant's inherited immune cells and those immune cell produce more virus instead of cleaning it up. This Trojan horse model of serious dengue can cause serious neurological defects in infants.

The neurological damage in infants from dengue has been well studied. Researchers have shown that infants whose mothers were infected with dengue who had previously been infected with another of the dengue types (remember, there are four) were far more likely to have serious side effects. The combination of two different Dengue infections explained 98% of serious dengue infant cases.

Since dengue and Zika virus are closely related, it seems possible that a previous or current dengue infection could help the Zika virus enter the brain of the infant and cause its destruction. Antibodies confused by the Zika virus would bind to it rather than to dengue and bring it into the immune cells to replicate, causing severe disease.

If that co-infection Trojan horse model explains even some of the cases of Zika microcephaly, then testing for high dengue antibody levels could show the increased risk of serious birth defects for pregnant mothers infected with Zika. Currently this is not being done, when it could differentiate between unborn children at high-risk vs. those at low risk for serious side effects.

While dengue is the most likely suspect for co-infection, other members of the flavivirus family could help trigger an "anamnesia" response resulting in a Trojan horse model of severe side effects. The area of northeastern Brazil reporting the most birth defects has previously suffered from widespread yellow fever. We also had the concurrent outbreak of Chikungunya virus in the same area, which also could have generated antibodies that acted as Trojan horses. In other words, the greatly increased number of microcephaly cases in Brazil may have been the perfect storm, not a repeatable event in other parts of the world.

8 GUILLAIN-BARRÉ SYNDROME

The other fear from Zika virus is that it causes Guillain-Barré Syndrome (GBS), an attack by the immune system on the nervous system as the result of the infection. GBS symptoms can range from tingling to difficulty breathing. While patients usually reach their weakest point about three weeks after they get GBS, they can remain weak for days and months later. The National Institutes of Health estimates that about one in three GBS patients has continuing weakness even three years later.

Given its dire nature and uncertain prognosis, GBS is almost more feared than Zika virus itself. The virus doesn't affect more than a few people with GBS, but cases of GBS found in active Zika areas are twice as likely to have been exposed to Zika virus.

Studies of brain tissue have also found that Zika attacks the nerves, but Zika alone doesn't seem to cause GBS. So far we've seen GBS cases skyrocket in areas where both dengue and Zika are circulating side-by-side. Patients with GBS had typically been exposed to both viruses.

An infection with any of the other flaviviruses might cause the same over-reaction by the body, the anamnesia response discussed in the last chapter. So during an co-occurring outbreak of dengue and Zika virus, victims may be mounting a dramatic attack on dengue when Zika virus infects them. That attack could worsen the normally milder symptoms, with the Trojan horse model of drawing in still-active Zika virus into the cells.

There is also another anamnesia response within the body that involves an autoimmune attack of the body on its own cells. Both Zika and dengue viruses share a number of common surface markers with the body's nerve cells. So if the body is desperately trying to rid itself of Zika by mistakenly using a dengue response, it may overreact. It might in desperation begin manufacturing antibodies that attack infected nerve cells directly rather than the freely circulating Zika virus. In other words, the body begins to damage its own nerves while trying to destroy the virus.

The case reports of Zika show that the most severe symptoms including GBS often occur just as the patient has mostly recovered from the virus. It's as if the body, recovering from the infection, suddenly goes into overdrive and makes the person much, much sicker.

The body may not be entirely mistaken in attacking its own infected cells. Remember that the Zika virus mutates, and some of those mutations could be faulty enough that they don't cause the nerve cell to explode with virus. Instead, the nerve cells may have the virus remain dormant within them, and some may even incorporate it into existing cell structures. Some experts theorize that much of our own DNA may be made up of acquired DNA we have incorporated from previous viral infections dating back to when we were much simpler organisms. But that incorporated Zika genetic material in the cell may trigger the immune system to attack the cells that contain it.

The best way to think about the serious state of a person with GBS is that they have an autoimmune disease triggered by a mistaken response to an infectious disease. That autoimmune response is most likely caused by a previous infection with a similar virus. So individuals getting Zika for the first time should be at much lower risk for Guillain-Barré Syndrome.

Focusing on Guillain-Barré as an autoimmune reaction rather than an side effect of infection means a change in possible treatment options. Treatments that might be effective for allergies or other autoimmune diseases (steroids, immunoglobulins) might be tried, particularly in chronic GBS patients who have not yet fully recovered.

How do you avoid Guillain-Barré Syndrome? You can't, but you can know that it's very likely that multiple exposures are necessary to set off the reaction, and that even with multiple exposures it's very rare.

9 HOW LONG DOES IT LAST?

According to the standard model of Zika virus, it is a rapid, violent illness that either resolves quickly or leads to rapid side effects. As such, long term monitoring of recovered Zika patients hasn't been done to determine if patients remain infectious.

Clearly, previously infected patients maintain immune memory cells for an extended time, possibly for life. This lifelong immunity does tend to deteriorate with age, so that the memory cells stop putting out as many antibodies and the antibodies have a decreased range of response. Over time the ability of the antibodies to attack similar viruses decreases, they become less flexible, more rigid in their abilities. Researchers think of this as a "brittle" immune response, and it may be part of the reason that older people have more serious side effects from Zika virus.

But how long is a person infectious? We don't know. The focus on mosquitoes means that no one has tracked Zika virus long term in humans. We do know that Zika virus remains in the semen of victims for at least two months, which is the longest anyone has tracked the infection.

But if we acknowledge that Zika may be similar to the West Nile flavivirus, then researchers have found West Nile virus in victims up to seven years after the initial infection. These individuals were not fully recovered. They had the severe nerve involvement of West Nile, and continued to have the nerve symptoms of the infection while dumping the virus in their body fluids.

It's a huge leap to go from seven days (the acute phase of Zika) to seven years (West Nile). But the little we know is that Zika virus patients also shed virus in their saliva at least a few weeks after getting better. If prolonged shedding is infectious, then you have a scenario where Zika virus would not only be spread by humans, it could be maintained by them. Mosquitoes, in that case, would be incidental to the continued spread of infection.

The reality may be that Zika virus only remains active for a short period around its acute infection state. Patients shedding viral material in their saliva and urine may not be able to infect other people. But, like other viral diseases, a subpopulation of those infected may become chronically infected with continuing symptoms (such as patients with ongoing GBS symptoms) and act as carriers to the rest of the population.

In the history of Zika, experts note long periods of silence. These periods are not explained by twenty year droughts or other losses of the mosquito population. The absence may be explained by the relative isolation of human carriers who later interact with the rest of the population and spark a new outbreak.

Currently, the concept of a chronic carrier has been confined to the monkey population. But Zika virus may not be limited to only primates. It may, like dengue, infect a range of animal species. In one review, Zika antibodies were found exotic animals like elephants, hippos, and wildebeest. But other species like goats, sheep, and rodents also had antibodies to the Zika virus. These animals are wide ranging and raise the possibility of non-human, non-mosquito spread of Zika virus. Since the initial studies on multiple species carrying Zika virus was done in 1968, with hindsight it is hard to understand how we've overlooked other possible routes of Zika spread except that it hasn't previously been on the radar as a global problem.

With a longer possible period of infection and a wider range of hosts, Zika may be far more common globally than we believed previously. Only now that we are fully aware of it will we start to track its true prevalence in the world population. And as we do we will likely find that it is, like other flaviviruses, endemic in many areas and continually infecting victims at low levels even during "silent" periods without epidemics.

10 CAN WE AVOID SERIOUS SIDE EFFECTS?

The obvious answer to avoiding the serious side effects of Zika has been: don't get bitten. Wear an entire suit of permethrin treated clothing (unwashed), and a hat with a mosquito net. That basic protective recommendation is still a great idea, since it greatly decreases both your chance of being bitten and your chances of having an unprotected romantic encounter with anyone who isn't into that particular "survival" look. But just maintaining that sort of protection is unlikely to be enough.

More recently the official answer to avoiding serious Zika involves not traveling to any region where Zika has been found and not engaging in vaginal, anal, or oral sex with anyone who's traveled in those regions recently. Pregnant women would likely be safest to not ever have unprotected sex with their partners during pregnancy. Since other flaviviruses pass through the breast milk, pregnant women should likely avoid unprotected sex while breastfeeding. At this point it seems reasonable to expand that warning against unprotected sex to everyone regardless of pregnancy status. If saliva is infectious, the rule against traveling might include the warning to avoid sharing food or kissing anyone from a Zika endemic area.

So if you're trying to avoid getting serious side effects from Zika by avoiding any possibility of Zika infection, then your life just got far more complicated and possibly more lonely.

Is it reasonable to expect to avoid any exposure to Zika virus?

Remember the previous statistics in this book. You may have already had Zika but never noticed. Eighty percent of you may get infected with Zika virus, and get no symptoms at all.

If you do get Zika and do have symptoms, it doesn't mean that you will get serious side effects. In the vast majority of those who get Zika and have symptoms, it really is no worse than a bad cold. Most babies (99%) born to Zika infected mothers do not have birth defects. The vast majority patients recover from Zika without GBS. Serious side effects from Zika have been so rare in the past that doctors never bothered to check for Zika at all.

The people who are at highest risk for serious Zika are found mostly in populations that have been previously been exposed to multiple flaviviruses. But even in people who've previously been exposed to dengue or one of the other flaviviruses, the previous infection could be helpful in the majority of Zika infected patients, speeding their recovery. Having a few antibodies to start fighting Zika may be better than starting with none.

Only if the initial immune response doesn't result in a complete cure, then the patient's own overactive immune system may cause serious Zika. That less-effective response not only draws resources away from fighting Zika, it also acts as a Trojan horse to allow still active Zika into the cells. It is in this population of the previously infected who only mount a partial immune response that we see almost all our patients with serious Zika side effects. Serious Zika might occur from Zika alone, but it seems far less likely. It may be so unlikely that we should focus our attention on those who have had multiple exposures rather than tracking Zika transmission alone.

So far we've seen the increased global transmission of Zika, which is terrifying. As Zika spreads, the chances of multiple exposures and higher levels of serious side effects also spreads.

But if we take a step back from that increased transmission to look at the risks of serious disease, the picture is more reassuring. Women exposed to Zika alone are at extremely low risk of passing on a birth defect to their infant. Only those who've had multiple exposures are at any significant risk, and that risk is currently at one percent. Antibody levels of other flaviviruses may indicate more accurately than an active Zika infection alone whether the infant is at risk of a serious Zika reaction. Since the infant is dependent on the immune system of the mother, tracking the mother's immune response would be adequate for both.

Beyond monitoring for multiple exposures during pregnancy, little can be done for GBS besides recommending against getting bitten a number of times by mosquitoes infected with different viruses. Except we know a great deal about how to deal with an immune system that has become overactive. The same drugs that prevent autoimmune disease may lessen the effects of GBS and lower the risk of long-term nerve effects. Treating GBS the way we would any allergic reaction might go a long way toward resolving this serious version of Zika

If you are exposed to Zika, everything that we know about avoiding a worsening viral illness comes into play. Sleep, diet, lifestyle, and supplements may all be helpful. Estimates based on the transmission of other viruses estimate that even a five percent variation in sleep quality can increase the risk of worsening symptoms. What the researchers really mean is that poor sleep and poor eating habits can lower the immune system so that it has to go into a noticeable full body response to deal with the virus. Other people can deal with the same virus without ever showing symptoms.

In most cases, the serious Zika symptoms do not show up until the body has almost healed from the initial infection. As the body recovers, it suddenly has a great many immune cells looking for trouble. If they see nerve tissue that looks like the Zika virus, that is when serious illness occurs. So individuals wishing to avoid serious Zika should take particular care at the end of their illness, just when they'd like to get up and get back to their lives.

11 WHAT IS THE FUTURE OF ZIKA VIRUS?

To answer the question of where Zika virus will be in the future, let's look at the history of one of its fellow flaviviruses, dengue. From a viral standpoint, dengue is a viral pandemic success (good for it, bad for us). Over the past thirty years, the number of dengue cases has increased. Not doubled or tripled. No. The cases have increased fifty times. Every year between fifty to one hundred million cases of dengue occur worldwide.

If we follow dengue back to 1927, it hit Greece. The cases the first year were mild and disappeared with cold weather as the mosquitoes died off. Then in 1928 there was an epidemic that struck more than half a million people in Greece. Severe side effects were common, and a number of people died. Some researchers claim there were two different strains of dengue, but others say the blood tests don't confirm a new strain. Whatever the cause of the epidemic, dengue then disappeared from Greece and Europe for decades until two cases were discovered in Nice, France in this century. But researchers going back and checking European blood samples found that, without any reported epidemic, around five percent of the French population was already immune to dengue. Another study in Croatia found that five percent of the inhabitants were also immune to dengue.

Getting back to Zika, it also has had periodic epidemics and then appears to disappear from the population for an extended time. But when researchers check blood samples, again about five percent of the population is immune to Zika virus.

If we look at the current epidemic, it can be hard to see any silver lining to the storm. But there may be. If we look back, we see that widespread epidemics can lead to an extended absence of the disease. Since so many people are being infected with Zika currently, this may be that last time we see a Zika epidemic in our lifetimes.

The previous focus on the mosquito-borne aspect of Zika transmission served a good purpose. It resulted in widespread spraying to get rid of mosquitoes. But we've realized that widespread spraying of chemicals isn't the best way to keep the rest of the animal kingdom alive. So we've stopped widespread global spraying and now need another disease prevention model to help us prevent Zika's spread. Recognizing that humans, not mosquitoes, spread the Zika virus may provide greater prevention possibilities today.

Since the virus is blood borne, expect to see other animals implicated in the spread of Zika virus in the future. Currently the virus may inhabit only certain mosquitoes, but mutation may allow it to reside in creatures like fleas or ticks. Expecting to avoid it because you've avoided mosquitoes is unlikely to give you the protection you'd like going forward.

At some point Zika may be listed correctly as a sexually transmitted disease, leading to wider screening and awareness in a younger population more likely to travel and be carriers of the virus. The behaviors that prevent Zika transmission are also those that prevent other sexually transmitted diseases, including Ebola (which just recently was found to be sexually transmissible after the standard quarantine period).

The association of Zika with pregnancy risks may have a

secondary damping effect on those trying to conceive in areas considered to be at risk for Zika. Not knowing if your partner has Zika, are you willing to try and conceive a child? We may see a decline in pregnancy rates in areas considered at-risk as a result. Hopefully the information about birth defects being related to co-infection will lessen some prospective parents' fears. The immediate response in Brazil has been a massive increase in abortions. At this point a Brazilian child exposed to Zika is much more likely to be aborted than it is to be born with any birth defects.

Going forward, have we emptied the rainforests and swamps of viruses? Oh, no. There are many more viruses. Here are two more viruses to watch for. If they are part of the next epidemic, you heard it here first. Mayaro virus, which looks a lot like dengue, has been on the move in areas near the Amazon rainforest. Wesselsbron virus, which infects sheep and mosquitoes, has also been confirmed in humans in South Africa. Either one of these could spread like Zika unless we change the way we think about "mosquito borne" viruses.

We live in a world where it's very easy to blame someone or something else for our behavior. By taking responsibility for our own actions, we can avoid contributing to the spread of Zika virus.

So, what should you do to avoid getting Zika?

1)   Don't get bitten by mosquitoes if you live near someone with Zika.

2)   Don't collect old tires (and if you must have some around, you may block the growth of mosquitoes by adding tea to the water).

3)   Don't swap body fluids with strangers. Have long term partners, use protection, and don't lose your mind if your partner gets

a mosquito bite.

If you're pregnant:

1)   Relax, because the chances of birth defects from Zika is very, very small. Even if you live in Brazil and get bitten regularly, your child has at least an 87% chance of not having microcephaly. Anywhere else in the world the risk from Zika is 1%.

2)   Avoid getting bitten.

3)   Avoid getting two different flaviviruses.

4)   Don't swap body fluids with strangers.

5)   Have your partner use protection until you've finished breastfeeding.

#####

ABOUT THE AUTHOR

Dr. Christopher Maloney, N.D., writes simple books about complex issues. He graduated from Swarthmore College, got his premedical diploma from Harvard, and his medical degree from the National College of Natural Medicine. Dr. Maloney has practiced family medicine in Maine for over a decade. He hopes that this book helps you to avoid unnecessary risks while lowering your overall fear of the Zika virus.

RESEARCH LINKS

Research to support this book was compiled from free medline sources and news reports. All research links can be found at Naturopathicmaine.com under the book title. Dr. Maloney welcomes questions via email.

OTHER BOOKS
By Dr. Maloney
Helping Your NF1 Child: A Parents' Guide To Neurofibromatosis
Tending Your Internal Garden
The Colon Cancer Diet
Your Vehicle For Life
Joint Hypermobility Syndrome

www.ingramcontent.com/pod-product-compliance
Lightning Source LLC
Chambersburg PA
CBHW071133280526
45787CB00003B/1272